THE

KETO

Diet

THE COMPLETE GUIDE

First Published in 2017 by Oakleigh Publishing

Copyright 2017 @ Eva La Rouge

All rights reserved.

The transmission, duplication or reproduction of any of the following work, including precise information, will be considered an illegal act. The legality extends to creating a secondary or tertiary copy of the work or a recorded copy and is only allowed with express written consent of the Publisher.

ISBN-13: 978-1979794305
ISBN-10: 1979794308

The information in the following pages is broadly considered to be a truthful and accurate account of facts, and as such any inattention, use or misuse of the information in question by the reader will render any resulting actions solely under their purview. There are no scenarios in which the publisher or the original author of this work can be in any fashion deemed liable for any hardship or damages that may befall them after undertaking information described herein.

Interior, Front and Back Cover Design by Oakleigh Publishing and Eva La Rouge.

Printed in the United States of America.

First Edition

CONTENTS

AUTHOR

i

ACKNOWLEDGEMENT

ii

MEASUREMENT CONVERSION TABLE

iii

INTRODUCTION

iv

PART I: KETO CLARITY

EVERYTHING ABOUT THE INSTANT POT

2

THE HISTORY OF THE KETO DIET

6

THE SCIENCE OF THE KETO DIET

8

THE BENEFITS AND SIDE EFFECTS OF THE KETO DIET

12

KETO DIETING PRINCIPLES

16

IS THE KETO DIET THE BEST DIET?

17

RECIPES

PART II: SOUPS

Bonny Bone Broth

19

Beautiful Broccoli Cheese Soup

21

Contest-Winning Cauliflower Soup

23

Creamy Chicken Kale Soup

25

Gorgeous Ground Beef & Veggie Soup

27

PART III: STEWS

Bountiful Beef Curry Stew

31

Lovely Lamb Stew

33

Perfect Pork Cheek Stews

35

Satisfying Spicy Brazilian Fish Stew

37

Succulent Stewed Chicken

39

PART IV: CHILIS

Classy Chili
43
Burly Beef Chili
45
Creative Chicken Chili Verde
47
Crisp Chorizo Chili
49
Succulent Smoky Bacon Chili
51
Tasty Texas Chili
53
Tingling Tomatillo Chili
55

PART V: BEEF

Best Beef Ribs
59
Blissful Balsamic Beef Roast
61
Melt-In-Your-Mouth Moroccan Beef
63
Autumn Asian Pot Roast
65

Buxom Beef Stroganoff
67
Cozy Corned Beef and Cabbage
69
Nimble Noodle Lasagna
71

PART VI: PORK

Feisty Frittata
75
Knockout Kalua Pork
77
Ravishing Ribs
79
Perfect Pork Roast
81
Phenomenal Pulled Pork
83
Buzzing BBQ Ribs
85
Terrific Tandoori Pork Ribs
87

PART VII: LAMB

Irresistible Indian Kheema
91

Luxurious Lamb Shanks
93
Relishing Rich Lamb
95

PART VIII: CHICKEN

Jolly Jerk Chicken
99
Ceremonious Chicken Masala
101
Godly Garlic Butter Chicken
103
Remarkable Rotisserie Chicken
105

PART IX: SEAFOOD

Chic Creamy Shrimp & Bacon
109
Splendid Shrimp with Coconut Milk
111

PART X: VEGETARIAN & VEGAN

Handsome Hard-Boiled Eggs
115

Magnificent Mashed Cauliflower
117
Super Spaghetti Squash in Garlic Sauce
119

PART XI: SAUCES

Busting Black Bean Dip
123
Succulent Southwestern Spicy Spinach Dip
125
Considerate Cheeseburger Dip
127

PART XII: DESSERTS

Awesome Almond Carrot Cake
131
Caring Coconut Almond Cake
133
Delicious Dark Chocolate Walnut Cake
135
Lovely Lemon Cheesecake
137
Thai Coconut Custard
139

AUTHOR

Eva La Rouge is a fitness coach, nutritionist and grandmother to two wonderful grandchildren, but has struggled with her weight for years. After graduating from New York University with a degree in Health and Nutrition, Eva discovered the Keto diet back in 2008, and now enjoys renewed confidence, health and well-being. When she is not busy teaching and looking after her two grandchildren, Eva works as a fitness instructor at her local gym in Santa Monica. It is here where she helps women lose weight by teaching them all about the Keto diet. She has especially taught her students how to successfully incorporate alcohol into their lives by discovering a 'must know' happy balance between drinking and dieting – the best of both worlds!

ACKNOWLEDGEMENT

"To my dearest Scott"

I would like to dedicate this book to my husband Scott, without whom I would certainly not be the confident woman I am today. I would like to say a big thank you to my doctor, Tim Renaldas. Without his advice, I would not have started the Keto diet when I did. I would also like to thank Sharon and Bill for all their support over the past eight years. I would like to give a shout out to Cindy from the WeightLossPro team, as well as Tom, Mike, Joshua and all the folks down at Bay View Gym. Without their help and support, I most certainly would not be the healthy, confident and happy woman I am today. Finally, I would like to thank my two wonderful grandchildren for being a source of inspiration in my life. Kudos to you all!

....Eva

CONVERSION

HANDY BAKING CONVERSIONS & EQUIVALENTS

BUTTER
1 STICK OF BUTTER = 8 TABLESPOONS = 1/2 CUP

4 STICKS OF BUTTER = 32 TABLESPOONS = 2 CUPS

1 LARGE EGG = 1 TABLESPOON YOLK = 2 TABLESPOONS WHITE

1 CUP = 5 LARGE EGGS = 5-6 MEDIUM EGGS = 7 SMALL EGGS

1 LEMON = 1-3 TABLESPOONS JUICE = 1-1 1/2 TEASPOONS ZEST

4 LARGE LEMONS = 1/4 CUP GRATED ZEST

INTRODUCTION

Have you failed losing weight? Are you in a constant battle between your hips and lips? Do you want to shed those extra pounds and be that confident, healthy and youthful person you see in the mirror? Maybe you just don't have the confidence or know how to achieve your weight loss goals? Fear no more! If you've been asking yourself these questions, there is one thing I ask you to do right here and right now: STOP! Take a deep breath. Hold it. Now clear your mind of all the things you might have read on this matter.

Who am I?

Hi there! I'm Eva La Rouge. For the best part of 8 years, I have been on a Keto diet, and have been teaching it to friends, family and students from all around the world – students of different ages, sizes, sexes and backgrounds. From my humble beginnings in South Carolina, to my house here in bustling California, dieting has brought happiness to my life. Back in 2008, my friends, Bill and Sharon, spent a lot of time in and out of hospital. Sharon had lost her child at the time, and had gained a lot of weight comfort eating to cope with her loss. In a sense, who could blame her? Over the months, she gained a couple of dress sizes, and her weight was becoming more of an issue. After having a string of counseling sessions, she could cope better with her loss to such a degree that she now looked towards focusing on herself again. She was determined to be that slim, healthy girl she was back when she and Bill first met each other – and she achieved this. One year later, by sticking to the Keto diet, she was 70lbs lighter. Her confidence was through the roof. She now works as a weight loss coach at her local gym in Santa Monica. The rest is history! At the time, I was also suffering a weight problem of my own, but my problem was a bit different to hers. I'm a wine girl at heart. I love my wine! I'm what you would call a bit of a wine connoisseur. Diet after diet, the Atkins, Paleo and Zone etc., and year after year, I was not seeing the results I wanted to see. I questioned why I wasn't achieving the results my friends were enjoying. This suddenly changed when I watched the movie '... First Do No Harm' starring Meryl Streep. In this movie, a young boy was treated for epilepsy by sticking to a ketogenic diet. A few weeks after watching this movie, I saw a couple of television advertisements talking about the benefits the Keto diet has for us ordinary folk. I thought 'That sure does sound good – almost too real to be true.' At my next doctor's appointment, I spoke to my doctor, Tim Renaldes, about starting the Keto diet. Although hesitate, he gave me the green light. After years of experimenting with a variety of different types of alcohol, it turns out, I was simply drinking too much of it! However, it was not the quantity of alcohol I was drinking that was the problem, but the type of alcohol instead. This is an importance distinction that I explain in this book. As I have come to understand over the years, not understanding this simple fact can result in dieting failure.

This Book

Without further ado, let's get down to business by discussing what's inside this book. My aim with this book is to provide you with over 50 Instant Pot ketogenic recipes, which I myself have not only benefit from, but also my many students too. You can find a variety of tasty Keto friendly recipes in the following categories:

- Chilis, Soups, Stews
- Sauces, Seafoods, Desserts
- Vegan & Vegetarian
- Beef,
- Pork,
- Lamb
- Chicken

Each recipe is hand selected from thousands to ensure two things:

- It is tasty
- It contains optimum Keto diet ratios of carbohydrates, proteins and fats.

By selecting recipes like this, you not only get to taste the very best the Keto diet has to offer, but you will also be optimizing your weight loss. In other words, you will lose weight in the fastest, healthiest and tastiest way possible!

To help you with your cooking, each recipe provides the following:

- Optimized Keto ratios: Carbohydrates, Protein and Fat. You should read the 'Book Guide section to find our more information about this.
- Nutritional content! Now, it would be very silly of me not to provide you with this vital information. We all know how important keeping track of our values is on the Keto diet!
- Clear and easy to read layout. Each recipe is designed in such a way as to make it easy for you, the reader, to follow a recipe on your own.

PART I

KETO CLARITY

"Ketosis is the body's backup plan for when dietary fuel is not available. It pulls fat from storage and converts it to energy. Ketones are the by-products."

EVERYTHING ABOUT THE INSTANT POT

The Instant Pot is the brand name for a programmable countertop multi-cooker. Specifically, the device itself is a single countertop appliance that can perform multiple functions. The instant pot ideally replaces the following:

- Slow Cooker
- Pressure Cooker
- Rice Cooker
- Steamer
- Sauté/Browning Pan
- Yogurt Maker
- Warming Pan

Did you forget to thaw out something for dinner? No problem-o. The Instant Pot can handle it. The instant pot can cook baked potatoes cook in minutes and they are so fluffy on the inside too – tasty! Also, it can cook veggies cook in about five minutes while also preserving their nutrients It's also a slow cooker too. Did you catch that – it's a slow cooker that doesn't boil over! When it's finished slow cooking, it goes to the warm setting. Your food doesn't continue to cook, instead the instant pot keeps it nice and warm!

Revolutionary...

This single appliance has changed the way I cook. Most days I use the Slow Cooker or Pressure Cooker features. Because of this, I spend less time in my kitchen and more time doing the things I love. My grocery basket is now filled with vegetables because the instant pot perfectly cooks them and while not destroying any of the nutrients.

Once a week, I cook up a batch of hardboiled eggs for a quick breakfast when I must take my grandchildren to school early in the morning. The sauté/browning feature means I can saute veggies and brown meat in a single pot before setting the slow cooker. I occasionally toss things in the pot and set the Warming feature. It will warm up your food and then keep it warm for hours. You could put frozen soup into the pot in the morning, set it on Warm, and have perfectly heated soup for dinner ten hours later. This single appliance has made cooking faster and more convenient. (Even my husband has taken to using it!) I love that I can cook steel-cut oats for breakfast in a fraction of the time it would take on the stovetop, make rice to go with a last-minute stir-fry is in minutes, and slow-cook a stew.

In fact, it's even taken the place of my slow cooker, which has since been moved out of the kitchen.

Is it Safe?

I bet you're wondering why I would want a pressure cooker. Don't they occasionally explode and leave sweet potatoes on the ceiling? Well, this is a not your grandmother's pressure cooker. It has several safety features that are electronically controlled. It is impossible to open the lid until the pressure has been released either naturally or manually.

Don'ts!

- DON'T pre-heat the cooker.
- DON'T bring the cooker to pressure on high heat.
- DON'T walk away from a very full or wide cooker right after you've adjusted the heat.

Instant Pot FAQs

1. What is an Instant Pot? Is it the same as a pressure cooker?

Yes, the Instant Pot is currently one of the most popular electric pressure cooker brands. It is a multi-functional cooker that has some extra functions compare to traditional stove-top pressure cookers.

2. Is it called an InstaPot or Instant Pot?

Many users call it InstaPot, IP, or IPPY. The correct name is Instant Pot, but call it whatever you like. In fact, some users even name their cookers.

3. Is it easy to cook with an Instant Pot?

There's a learning curve to cook with pressure cookers. But no worries! Once you're familiar with it, you will find the cooking relatively easy.

4. Does the Instant Pot really speed up the cooking process?

Cooking in any pressure cooker is almost always faster. Tender and juicy pulled pork can be done in under 90 minutes, when it usually takes 2 – 4 hours to make in the oven.

5. Are there any disadvantages with cooking in the Instant Pot?

One disadvantage about cooking with any pressure cooker is you can't inspect, taste, or adjust the food along the way. That's why it's essential to follow recipes with accurate cooking times (like those recipes in this book).

6. Is Instant Pot safe to use?

Modern day electric pressure cookers like the Instant Pot are quiet, safe and easy to use. It has 10 UL Certified proven safety mechanisms to prevent most of the potential issues.

7. What is instant pot's working pressure?

The working pressure is in the range of 10.15~11.6 psi.

8. Can instant pot be used for pressure canning?

This is a direct quote from instant pot's official website: "instant pot has not been tested for food safety in pressure canning by USDA. We wouldn't recommend using instant pot for pressure canning purpose.

9. Can I use the Instant Pot for Pressure Frying?

Please don't attempt to pressure fry in any electric pressure cookers. The splattering oil may melt the gasket. KFC uses a commercial pressure fryer (modern ones operate at 5 PSI) specially made to fry chickens. This Pressure Cooker Chicken in this book is probably as close as it gets.

10. How to do a Quick Release?

After the cooking cycle ends, carefully move the venting knob from sealing position to venting position. This rapidly releases the pressure in the pressure cooker. This usually takes a few minutes. Wait until the floating valve (metal pin) completely drops before opening the lid.

11. How to do a Natural Release?

After the cooking cycle ends, wait until the floating valve (metal pin) completely drops before opening the lid. Always turn the venting knob from sealing position to venting position. This ensures all the pressure is released before opening the lid. It usually takes 10 – 25 minutes.

In these recipes, you may see "15 mins Natural Release" – this means after the cooking cycle ends, wait 15 minutes before turning the venting knob to manually release the remaining pressure.

THE HISTORY OF THE KETO DIET

The Early Days

To get a handle on the Keto diet, I find that the best place to start is always at the beginning. In this case, history shows us that in the 1920s and 1930s, the Keto diet was used as a treatment for patients with epilepsy. This was the only help sufferers had until medications were developed in later years. An interesting fact is that, in 20% to 30% of all cases, the Keto diet remained more effective than medications in treating epilepsy. Today, despite our medical advancements, the diet is still used as an alternative remedy to treat it, as well as providing other health benefits discussed later in this book.

In 1921, an by the name of Rollin Woodyatt, discovered that the diet helped our body in a remarkable way. It helped our liver produce three water-soluble compounds. These were:

1. β-hydroxybutyrate
2. acetoacetate
3. acetone

Accordingly...

Together, these compounds are known as ketone bodies. During the early 20th Century, an American by the name of Bernarr Macfadden, put forward fasting as a means of improving health. His student osteopath, Hugh Conklin, introduced fasting as a treatment for controlling epilepsy.

Coklin proposed that epileptic seizures were caused by a toxin secreted in the intestine and suggested that fasting for 18 to 25 days could cause the toxin to dissipate. His epileptic patients were put on a "water diet," which he reported cured 90% of children with the condition and 50% of adults. Analysis of the study that was performed later showed that, in fact, 20% of Coklin's patients became seizure-free, while 50% demonstrated some improvement. The fasting therapy was soon adopted as part of mainstream therapy for epilepsy and in 1916, Dr McMurray reported to the *New York Medical Journal* that he had successfully treated epileptic patients by prescribing a fast, followed by a diet free of starch and sugar since 1912.

The 1960s

Later, Russel Wilder, a medical student at the time coined the phrase 'ketogenic diet' for its use in the treatment of epilepsy. After considerable research in the 1960s, scientists found that medium-chain triglycerides produce even more ketones per unit of energy. This led to a revised Keto diet for epilepsy sufferers that was drawn up by Peter Huttenlocher. Here, 60 percent of a patient's daily calorie intake now came in the form of MCT oil.

Today

A larger variety of meals were now available for sufferers, and thus the Keto diet was born. And now we have the history behind the diet, let's take a look at it more closely. This was a significant discovery because it meant that patients could eat more carbohydrates and proteins, which lead to the possibility of a varied diet.

THE SCIENCE OF THE KETO DIET

In a nutshell, the Keto diet is a low carbohydrate diet. The intention behind it is for your body to produce ketones as a source of energy. This happens when your body gets into a state called ketosis. This is achieved by eating fewer carbs (5% - 10%), more fat (60% - 75%) and moderate protein (15% - 30%).

What is Ketosis?

"Ketosis is the body's backup plan for when dietary fuel is not available. It pulls fat from storage and converts it to energy. Ketones are the by-products."

Normally, our bodies process the carbohydrate we eat on an average balanced diet by turning it into glucose for energy.

When ketosis is reached, our body begins to use the ketones produced from the transfer of fat to energy. If ketosis is maintained, our body can enter a metabolic state where it will continue to burn these ketones. Ketosis is not a foreign process for our body. It happens naturally when our glucose levels are low. As we have seen, this can help treat epilepsy, but can also help us optimize our weight loss goals, as well as improving our overall confidence and well-being. This process also helps improve our body's resistance to insulin, and so is often an excellent choice for diabetics. We mentioned ketones, but what exactly are they? When our body breaks down fat for energy, certain byproducts are produced. These are known as ketone bodies or ketones for short. The process works as follows:

- When our body doesn't have enough glucose, our glycogen levels will eventually run out.
- Our body now begins to burn fuel differently since the glycogen stores are now gone.
- It does this by using fat to fuel itself.
- Once the body uses fat for energy, which is known as beta-oxidation, our liver will start to produce ketones that fuel our entire system.
- When our body reaches this state, it is said to be in ketosis.
- This produces three types of ketone bodies produced:

1. β-hydroxybutyrate
2. acetoacetate
3. acetone

Our metabolism is happy burning carbohydrates for fuel. Simple sugars from bread, rice, and sweets are broken down with little thought or energy, providing enough fuel to get through the day. If provided steady sources of carbohydrate throughout the day, things run smoothly. The problem is unless we are giving our bodies only what it needs for carbohydrates, the rest of those simple sugars will be stored as fat to use later, perhaps if you miss a meal. Weight gain happens when we consistently eat more than our bodies need to survive at any given time. Physiologically speaking, this is necessary, so we don't keel over between meals, but these days, inactivity plus huge portions mean we will keep storing fuel we don't intend to burn – we gain weight.

When we do not have a source of steady carbohydrates during the day, our metabolism shifts to pull fat from our stores, and burn it for energy. This fat-burning process is called ketosis, and the byproduct of this is ketones. Ketosis is the body's natural back up to burning carbohydrates as a matter of survival. As you could imagine, ketosis helps us lose weight because we are constantly burning fat for fuel instead of burning carbs as they come into the system. The problem is, it takes a bit of time to enter ketosis, and as soon as we eat carbohydrates, the body goes back to burning sugars. We can build our diets around proteins and fats instead of carbohydrates to mimic carbohydrate starvation to push our bodies into ketosis. While everyone will be a little bit different, the threshold of carbohydrates is about 50-60 grams per day, and about 10-15 grams per meal, before we exit ketosis. To put this into perspective, 15 grams is equal to a small slice of bread. To make the most of the meals, most of these carbs will be in sources like vegetables with low carb content. The basic ketogenic meal is a combination of proteins like chicken and fish, with a large side of non-starchy vegetables like salad and zucchini. Fats can be used without real restriction as well, so healthy fats like olive oil and avocado can be used to make up for the calories not taken up by carbohydrate-rich starches like rice and potato. Here is a brief list of what is allowed on the Keto diet:

Proteins	Vegetables
Chicken	Lettuce
Fish	Tomato
Beef	Spinach
Pork	Green beans
Turkey	Zucchini
Eggs	Cabbage/Cole slaw

Overeating any of these vegetables could set you over your carbohydrate goal, so make sure to keep track of grams of carbohydrate per serving. Keep in mind that you can also have starchier vegetables like broccoli and carrots in smaller portions. Use online resources for lists of common food carb contents and apps like MyFitnessPal to track total carb intake. If you have been a good guinea pig and following the rules, how do you know if you are in ketosis? Recent advances in science have developed test strips to test urine for ketones. A small number of ketones will be flushed out of the system in urine during ketosis, so if they are present in your urine, you are in ketosis. Testing regularly throughout the process can help you gauge just how high your carbohydrate tolerance is.

The 50-60gram guideline is just that, a guideline. Some people will enter ketosis at higher or lower levels of carbs, making testing necessary. Like any good diet, there must be some sort of calorie goal. Any type of food in excess will be stored as fat for later use. With the Keto diet, the food options are limited mainly to proteins and vegetables, which are naturally low calorie. It will likely be difficult to even max out your calories, but it is important to stay within a good range to maintain calories. The average active person will need somewhere between 1600 and 2200 calories daily depending on age, sex current weight and activity level. It may feel like you are eating too much food, but vegetables are low calorie, so it is very easy to under eat on a Keto plan. Use the guide in part III of this book to help make your meal plan.

THE BENEFITS AND SIDE EFFECTS OF THE KETO DIET

Weight Loss

Weight loss is arguably the most beneficial benefit of the Keto diet. When you reach a state of ketosis, your body burns fat to produce ketones. In many respects, your body is much like a machine. It burns fat in the most efficient way possible by tapping into your fat reserves all around your body – but cannot spot reduce! As you progress further into the Keto diet, you might notice that you can concentrate and focus on tasks more effectively than you could before. There is plenty of scientific evidence to suggest that. as your body reaches a state of ketosis, your brain receives and uses more ketones.

These ketones have been scientifically proven to be responsible for controlling your ability to concentrate. In fact, lots of people who are in physically decent shape use the Keto diet to improve their mental performance. There is a common misconception that, for your brain to function properly, it requires a certain amount of carbohydrates. This gives some people the impression that, as the Keto diet is about limiting carbohydrate intake, it is may reduce your mental performance. This is not true. After around 1-2 weeks of your brain adapting to the Keto diet, it uses the supply of ketones that are increasing available – this increases your mental performance.

What tends to confuse people is that, before your brain adapts to this, you may suffer from side effects – symptoms of the Keto diet. This might be a headache, common cold, and difficulty concentrating. You must understand that, once your body has adapted and overcome this 'adaption' stage, you can enjoy the benefits that the Keto diet offers: higher energy levels, concentration, mood and overall mental health.

Improved Physical Endurance

As you progress further into the Keto diet, you might notice your physical endurance improve. There is a lot of scientific research to suggest that, as a Keto diet accesses all the energy stored in your fat reserves, it can improve your physical endurance. Most people's bodies aren't using all this energy because not all their fat stores are available, especially if they eat a diet high in carbohydrates. Your body's ability to burn these carbohydrates (or glycogen) is limited to only a few hours when you're physically active, especially if you're working out. This might make you feel like eating before and after a workout, if you've been out walking, or even doing day to day chores like housekeeping. The keto diet solves this problem because, by restricting your carbohydrate intake, your body taps into energy stored in your fat reserves to feed your brain the vital ketones it needs.

A Treatment for Diabetes

Another benefit of the Keto diet is that it is a low carbohydrate diet. There is a lot of scientific research to suggest that the diet is an excellent remedy for controlling, or even reversing type II diabetes.

As you might know already, a high blood sugar level is a main factor in causing diabetes. For most people, the source of this sugar comes from the carbohydrates they eat. As the Keto diet is about limiting the carbohydrates you eat, it should be no surprise that the less of them you eat, the lower your blood sugar will be. This decrease in blood sugar is a natural benefit the Keto diet provides. However, as a word of caution, if you are a diabetic and want to start the Keto diet, you should speak to your doctor about your medications because you may have to adjust the amount you take to balance out this process. Perhaps the most common side effect of the Keto diet, and one which I have personally experienced, is the Keto flu. When your body transitions to burning ketones, you may experience a few troublesome symptoms.

The most common ones are: nausea, mood swings, muscle cramps and poor overall wellbeing. Personally speaking, nausea affected me the most when I made the transition. I know people who suffered a lot, and others who didn't suffer at all. What symptoms you have depends on your body and its ability to adapt to this change – don't worry though, as you will recover eventually! There are a few things you can do to make this transition go more smoothly.

- <u>Gradually</u> reduce your carbohydrate intake. body is a machine and takes time to adjust. Allow time for the ketones to kick it. Create a meal plan that allows you to reduce your intake gradually over a few weeks to a month. In the meantime, drink a cup of bouillon to help alleviate these symptoms.

Bad Breath

This is probably going to be the most unwanted and embarrassing side effect for you. Bad breath is produced by acetone, which is a type of ketone your body produces during ketosis. It smells quite like bleach or cleaning fluid – an unpleasant smell you certainly don't want! Drinking alcohol can make this smell even worse too. Despite this, it is a positive thing because it tells you that your body is in a state of ketosis. I know people who suffered from bad breath a lot during the first few months, and others who didn't suffer at all. Whether you suffer from it depends on your body and its ability to adapt to this change – don't worry though, as you will recover eventually! Excellent oral hygiene is yet to preventing bad breath, so make sure you always carry around some dental spray, floss and gum.

Loss of Fluids

Some changes in the amount of bodily fluids in your body might occur when you start the Keto diet. Don't worry! These changes are totally normal and happen as your body uses up its sugar (glycogen) stores. These stores release water into your blood, which passes out of your body as urine. As fluid is passed out of your body, your bodily salts may deplete too. As a result, you may experience a loss of fluid and salts as you move into and maintain ketosis. To remedy this problem, I find that keeping hydrated throughout the day works just fine. Water is the best drink for staying hydrated, but tea and coffee are equally as good, provided they're not too milky (milk is not Keto friendly)! If you are eating healthy and natural foods (such as nuts, meat, fish, dairy), you shouldn't have a problem!

DIETING PRINCIPLES

The Do's

- Your daily calories should come from: carbohydrates 5% - 10%, fat 60% - 75% and protein 15% - 30%.
- You should not eat more than 50g of carbohydrates daily.
- You should try to eat monounsaturated fats, saturated fats and omega oils,
- You should not eat fruit and other snacks when you are close to your carb limit.
- You should not starve yourself – eat when you are hungry. Starving yourself long term is a path to failure.
- You should not eat processed foods.
- You should stock up non-starchy vegetables, eggs, avocado, meat and other fermented foods like tuna fish – you never know what disaster might prevent your next trip to the grocery store!
- You should not eat vegetable soils, hydrogenated oils, margarine, trans fat, soybean and corn oil.
- You should eat raw and organic dairy products like unpasteurized milk, not pasteurized milk.
- You should be wary of food packing that says 'fat-free' because these may contain hidden fats and salt.
- You should eat salmon, nuts and avocados to avoid an electrolyte deficiency.

WHY IS THE KETO DIET BETTER THAN OTHER DIETS?

Now that's an interesting question. Why? Well in some cases, the difference between certain diets and the Keto diet is as big as day and night. In other cases, there are diets fairly like it, but with minor differences here and there.

Let's look at a Keto diet again before we compare. The ratios of carbohydrates/fat/protein taken in daily are:

- Carbohydrates 5%-10%
- Fat 60% - 75%
- Protein 15% - 30%

Now let's compare this with other diets.

The Keto Diet Vs a Balanced Diet

Although a balanced diet might vary amongst nutritional experts, it is usually broken down as follows:

- Carbohydrates 45% to 65%
- Fat 20% to 35%
- Protein 10% to 30%

The Keto Diet Vs the Paleo Diet

With the Paleo diet, the ratio of carbohydrates, protein, and fat is as follows:

- Carbohydrates 22% to 40%
- Fat 28% to 47%
- Protein 19% to 35%

The Keto Diet Vs the Zone Diet

The popular Zone diet has the following macronutrient ratios:

- Carbohydrates 40%
- Fat 30%
- Protein 30%

The Keto Diet Vs the Atkins Diet

When looking at the macronutrient ratios for the Atkins diet, you can see they are similar to those of the Keto diet.

- Carbohydrates 5%
- Fat 60%
- Protein 35%

To determine your individual calorie needs, use a trusted online calculator or consult with a doctor or registered dietitian. The good news is, it takes a ton of non-starchy vegetables to exceed calories, so you will likely be overstuffed before that ever happens. If you can be disciplined enough to maintain ketosis for good stretches of time, the diet will help you lose weight.

Most people fail in this discipline, adding in carbohydrates that quickly pull them back to burning them for fuel. Once ketosis is entered, the body doesn't really crave any carbohydrates, but getting over that hump can be difficult. Stick to your guns, get over carbohydrates and lose weight with ketosis.

PART II
SOUPS

Soups are a great dish that can be used in virtually any season. They are especially tasty in the cooler months, though, when they can help you warm up with a hearty dish while still being nutritious and contributing to your health goals. In this section, we will explore a few of the best ketogenic-friendly soups that you can make in your instant pot.

BONE BROTH

This recipe needs 5 minutes to prepare, 60 minutes to cook, and will make 12 cups.

- Protein: 3.6g
- Net Carbs: 0.7g
- Fats: 6g
- Calories: 72

The macronutrient ratio of this meal is: 4% carbs, 20.2% protein, and 75.8% fat.

Ingredients:

- Chicken Carcass (1 cooked, nearly meatless)
- Celery Tops (1 C or 250mL)
- Ginger (1 inch)
- Garlic (2 cloves)
- Onion (1, quartered)
- Filtered Water (3L)
- Apple Cider Vinegar (2 T)

INSTRUCTIONS

1. Begin by placing all your ingredients in your instant pot. Top it off with water until it reaches the 4L mark.
2. Seal instant pot and manually set it to high pressure. Set the timer for 60 minutes.
3. When it has completely cooked, allow your instant pot to naturally release the pressure. Allow it to cool for 60 minutes before removing it from the instant pot.
4. Once cooled, strain the broth into a large, sealable container. Seal the container and place in the fridge overnight.
5. In the morning, scrape the fat that has solidified on the top of the broth. Discard it, then separate broth into containers to be easily used as needed.
6. Store your bone broth in an air tight container for up to 1 week in your refrigerator or for up to 3 minutes in your freezer.

BROCCOLI CHEESE SOUP

This recipe needs 5 minutes to prepare, 5 minutes to cook, and it will create enough soup for 4 servings.

- Protein: 5.6g
- Net Carbs: 1g
- Fats: 30g
- Calories: 350g

The macronutrient ratio of this meal is: 5% carbs, 7% protein, and 19% fat.

Ingredients:

- Broccoli (1 large bunch, florets only)
- Sharp Cheddar (2 C or 500mL, shredded)
- Heavy Cream (1 C or 250mL)
- Chicken Stock (4.C or 1000mL)
- Onion Powder (1 T)
- Garlic Powder (.25 TSP)
- Butter (2 T)
- Shredded Carrots (1 C or 250mL)

INSTRUCTIONS

1. Brown the butter in your instant pot over medium heat. Once melted, add remaining ingredients, except for heavy cream and cheese, to the instant pot. Secure lid in place and cook on high for 5 minutes.
2. Complete a quick release of the steam according to your manufacturers standards before removing the lid.
3. Stir in heavy cream and cheese now until cheese is fully melted, and soup is smooth and creamy.
4. Serve & Enjoy!

CAULIFLOWER SOUP

This recipe needs 20 minutes to prepare, 5 minutes to cook, and it will create enough soup for 4-6 servings.

- Protein: 10.7g
- Net Carbs: 1g
- Fats: 19.1g
- Calories: 251

The macronutrient ratio of this meal is: 5% carbs, 17.6% protein and 70.9% fat.

What to Use:

- Cauliflower (1 large head, coarsely chopped)
- Cheddar Cheeses (1 C or 250mL, grated)
- Chicken Stock (3 C or 750mL)
- Butter (2 T)
- Onion (.5, chopped)
- Garlic Powder (1 TSP)
- Salt (1 TSP)
- Half and Half (.5C or 125mL)
- Cream Cheese (4oz)

INSTRUCTIONS

1. Begin by preparing your vegetables to be cooked. When done, turn your instant pot to the "sauté" mode so that you can brown your butter. Allow the butter to melt completely before sautéing your onions to a translucent color.
2. Add remaining ingredients except for dairy products. Manually set your instant pot to high pressure and cook for 5 minutes before performing the quick release method as outlined by your manufacturer's manual.
3. Stir in dairy products now, continuing to stir until they blend in smoothly. Transfer ingredients to a blender and blend until the soup is completely pureed. If you do not have a high-power blender, you could also use a food processor. If it has become too thick, add more chicken stock.
4. Serve.

CHICKEN KALE SOUP

This recipe needs 5 minutes to prepare, 15 minutes to cook, and it prepares enough soup for 4 servings.

- Protein: 1.7g
- Net Carbs: 0.9g
- Fats: 14.4g
- Calories: 154

The macronutrient ratio of this meal is: 4% carbs, 4% protein, and 82% fat.

Ingredients:

- Carrots (1 C or 250mL, peeled and cubed)
- Onion (1.5 cups or 375mL, chopped)
- Butter (2 T)
- Celery (1 C or 250mL)
- Chicken Breast (2 C or 500mL, cooked and shredded)
- Kale (2 C or 500mL, chopped)
- Bay Leaves (2 whole)
- Salt (1 TSP)
- Thyme (.5 TSP)
- Oregano (.25 TSP)
- Black Pepper (0.5 TSP)
- Chicken Broth (4 C or 1000mL)
- Worcestershire Sauce (.5 TSP)
- Water to top

INSTRUCTIONS

1. Begin by melting your butter on the "sauté" function in your instant pot so that you can sauté your onions until they are translucent. Add remaining vegetables and spices and cook until you can smell the aromas well.
2. Add chicken broth and top with water until instant pot is filled to the 6-cup line.
3. Cancel sauté function and transfer to soup function, or to high pressure mode. Cook for 4 minutes before conducting a manual pressure release as per your manufacturer's instructions. Remove the lid and add kale and chicken to the instant pot. Allow to settle for about 1 minute before adding salt, Worcestershire sauce, and pepper.
4. Serve.

GROUND BEEF & VEGGIE SOUP

This recipe needs 5 minutes to prepare, 50 minutes to cook, and will prepare enough soup for 4-6 servings.

- Protein: 34.9g
- Net Carbs: 8.4g
- Fats: 38.4g
- Calories: 520g

The macronutrient ratio for this meal is 6% carbs, 27% protein, and 67% fat.

INGREDIENTS:

- Olive Oil (1 TSP)
- Onion (1 C or 250mL, chopped)
- Ground Beef (1lb)
- Garlic (1 T, minced)
- Thyme (1 TSP)
- Green Beans (1 C or 250mL, ends trimmed and cut into bite sized pieces)
- Oregano (1 TSP)
- Diced Tomatoes with Juice (2 Cans, 15oz each)
- Beef Broth (3.5 C or 875mL)

INSTRUCTIONS

1. Begin by turning your instant pot to the sautéing function so that you can brown your butter. When butter is melted, cook beef until it has browned thoroughly. Break it apart as it cooks so it does not remain in chunks.
2. Add chopped onion to your instant pot, as well as garlic and spices. Cook until the garlic is fragrant, and the onions have softened.
3. Add tomatoes with juice and broth, allowing them to heat in the pressure cooker for a few minutes before adding your beans.
4. Seal lid and cook for 30 minutes on low pressure setting. Quick release your lid to remove the soup and serve hot.

PART III
STEWS

If you are looking for something a little more filling but still healthy, stews are a great option! These dishes are filled with nutritious elements such as chunky meats and keto-friendly vegetables, and warm gravy to add to the taste and texture of the meal. These are just like the ones you always crave during those cold months, only they honor your ketogenic requirements!

BEEF CURRY STEW

This recipe needs 5 minutes to prepare, 50 minutes to cook, and it will prepare enough stew for 6 servings.

- Protein: 40g
- Net Carbs: 8g
- Fat: 30g
- Calories: 490

The macronutrient ratio for this meal is 6% carbs, 31% protein, and 62% fat.

INGREDIENTS:

- Beef Stew Chunks (2.5lb)
- Curry Powder (2 TBSP)
- Broccoli Florets (2 C or 500mL)
- Zucchini (3 C or 750mL, chopped)
- Chicken Broth (0.5 C or 125mL)
- Coconut Milk (14oz)
- Garlic Powder (1 TBSP)

INSTRUCTIONS

1. Combine all ingredients except coconut in instant pot and give a good mix. Manually set your instant pot to the high pressure setting and cook the stew for 45 minutes. Then, perform a quick release based on your instant pot's manufacturer's manual.
2. Stir in coconut milk, season to desired taste.
3. Serve.

LAMB STEW

This recipe needs 5 minutes to prepare, 35 minutes to cook, and will prepare enough stew to make 4 servings.

- Protein: 35.9g
- Net Carbs: 1.1g
- Fats: 46.5g
- Calories: 583

The macronutrient ratio of this recipe is 0.74% carbs, 24.9% protein, and 74.3% fat.

INGREDIENTS

- Acorn Squash (Peeled, Seeds Removed, Cubed)
- Lamb Stew Meat (2lbs)
- Carrots (1.5 C or 375mL)
- Onion (1 C or 250mL, cut into 1" slices)
- Garlic (6 cloves, sliced)
- Bay (1 Leaf)
- Broth (3 T)
- Rosemary (1-2 sprigs)

INSTRUCTIONS

1. Begin by preparing your acorn squash, slicing your carrots, and cubing your onions. When done, add all your ingredients into your pressure cooker.
2. Manually set instant pot to the high pressure setting and cook your lamb stew for 35 minutes. When the stew is done, execute a quick release on your pressure as described in your owner's manual for your instant pot.
3. Serve.

PORK CHEEK STEWS

This recipe needs 5 minutes to prepare, 55 minutes to cook, and will make enough to serve 6-8 bowls of stew.

- Protein: 39.2g
- Net Carbs: 8.6g
- Fats: 39.2g
- Calories: 571

The macronutrient ratio for this recipe is 6% carbs, 29% protein, and 65% fat.

INGREDIENTS

- Pork Cheek (4lb cut into 1-inch slices)
- Avocado Oil (2 T)
- Pork Broth (1.5 C or 375mL)
- Cremini Mushrooms (1 cup or 250mL)
- Leek (1 C or 250mL, cut into .5-inch chunks)
- Onion (.5 cup or 125mL, diced)
- Lemon Juice (1 T)
- Garlic (6 cloves, peeled)

INSTRUCTIONS

1. Turn instant pot to sear setting and sear pork cheeks. Work in batched until all pieces have been seared on each side.
2. Cover with broth and add remaining ingredients. Cook for 45 minutes using "meat and stew" setting.
3. Using manufacturer's instructions, perform a quick release on your instant pot and remove pork from the pot. Set it on a cutting board so you can shred it to bite-sized pieces. Transfer remaining ingredients to a blender and blend until smooth and creamy.
4. Return shredded meat to broth and serve immediately.

SPICY BRAZILIAN FISH STEW

This recipe needs 10 minutes to prepare, 20 minutes to cook, and will make enough for 2 servings.

- Protein: 36.9g
- Net Carbs: 2g
- Fats: 36.9g
- Calories: 530

The macronutrient ratio for this recipe is 2% carbs, 30% protein, and 68% fat.

INGREDIENTS

- White Fish (1 pound, any kind)
- Lime Juice (1 TSP)
- Jalapeno Pepper (1 T, seeds removed and diced)
- Red Pepper (1 C or 250mL, diced)
- Yellow Pepper (1 C or 250mL, diced)
- Onion (1 C or 250mL, diced)
- Garlic (2 cloves, minced)
- Chicken Broth (2 C or 500mL)
- Tomatoes (2 C or 500mL, chopped)
- Paprika (1 TSP)
- Coconut Milk (15oz can)
- Olive Oil (1 T)

INSTRUCTIONS

1. Marinate fish in lime juice as you prepare remaining ingredients in recipe.
2. While fish marinates, turn instant pot to sauté function and allow it to heat your oil until it begins to sizzle. Then, go ahead and add your diced vegetables into your instant pot. Allow the vegetables to cook until they soften. Add garlic and continue cooking until garlic becomes fragrant.
3. Add remaining ingredients except for fish and coconut milk. Stir well then boil.
4. Add fish and coconut milk, stirring thoroughly. Manually set instant pot to medium pressure and cook for 10 minutes. Fish should be completely cooked before removing from the pot. It will be flaky when it is done.
5. Serve.

STEWED CHICKEN

This recipe needs 5 minutes to prepare, 30 minutes to cook, and it will prepare enough stew to serve about 8 servings.

- Protein: 31.9g
- Net Carbs: 9.1g
- Fats: 48.6g
- Calories: 639

The macronutrient ratio of this recipe is 6% carbs, 21% protein, and 73% fat.

INGREDIENTS

- Chicken Legs (4 whole, separate thighs from drumsticks)
- White Vinegar (2 T)
- Coconut oil (1 T)
- Recado Rojo Paste (2 T)
- Garlic (3 cloves, sliced)
- Worcestershire Sauce (3 T)
- Ground Cumin (1 TSP)
- Chicken Stock (2 C or 500mL)
- Dried Oregano (1 TSP)
- Onion (1 C or 250mL, sliced)
- Optional: Granulated Sugar Substitute (such as erythritol) (1 T)

INSTRUCTIONS

1. In a large bowl mix together pepper, cumin, oregano, recado paste, vinegar, Worcestershire sauce, and optional sweetener. Blend thoroughly and use to marinate chicken. Allow to marinate overnight, or at least for 1 hour.
2. Turn instant pot to sauté mode and heat coconut oil. Once hot, cook chicken in batches so you can brown the skin. Do this for approximately 2 minutes per side. Keep remaining marinade in the bowl for later.
3. Sauté garlic and onions for 3 minutes. Add chicken back into pot.
4. In bowl with marinade, mix in broth and stir well to combine marinade and broth before pouring it into the instant pot.
5. Seal instant pot and manually set to high pressure so it can cook for 20 minutes. Using manufacturer's instructions, perform a quick release.
6. Serve.

PART IV
CHILLI

Chilies are another great dish that can be eaten as is poured over top of ketogenic friendly vegetables to make an even more filling dish. There are many incredibly delicious and nutritious chilies you can make that honor your diet, which you will find in this chapter.

CHILI

This recipe needs 5 minutes to prepare, 30 minutes to cook, and it will prepare enough stew to serve about 1 serving.

- 318 Calories
- 30.91g Protein
- 18.99g Fats
- 6g Net Carbs

The macronutrient ratio of this recipe is 3% carbs, 16% protein, and 81% fat.

INGREDIENTS

- 1 tbsp salT
- 2 tbsp Worcestershire saucE
- 14 oz/400g can whole tomatoes, drained
- 4 tbsp/60ml chopped pickled jalapenos
- 5 1/3 oz/150g chopped celery
- 4 cloves minced garlic
- 1 chopped onion
- 2 lbs/900g ground beef
- 3 tbsp olive oil
- 3 tbsp taco seasoning

INSTRUCTIONS

1. Cook ground beef with oil in a skillet with seasonings until no longer pink. Stir well to combine everything.

2. Put in the slow cooker.

3. Add remaining ingredients. Stir well. Tomatoes need to be drained well.

4. Cover. Set on low for six hours.

5. Taste and adjust seasonings, if needed.

6. Serve on low-carb tortillas with toppings of choice.

BEEF CHILI

This recipe needs 5 minutes to prepare, 30 minutes to cook, and will prepare enough chili for 4 servings.

- Protein: 39.1g
- Net Carbs: 6.1g
- Fats: 41.9g
- Calories: 570

The macronutrient ratio for this recipe is 5% carbs, 28.5% protein, and 66.5% fat.

INGREDIENTS

- Ground Beef (1lb)
- Onion (.5 Cup or 125mL, chopped)
- Red Pepper (1 Cup or 250mL, diced)
- Salt (.75 TSP)
- Ground Cumin (1 TSP)
- Black Beans (15oz can, rinsed)
- Garlic Powder (.25 TSP)
- Tomato Sauce (.5 cup or 125mL)
- Diced Tomatoes with Green Chilies (10oz can, drained)
- Broth (.75 C or 190mL)
- Chili Powder (.5 TSP)
- Paprika (.5 TSP)

INSTRUCTIONS

1. Sauté your beef in your instant pot until completely browned. Break it apart as you sauté it.
2. Cook onion and pepper until onion becomes translucent.
3. Add tomatoes, spices, broth and beans. Cover and cook by manually setting to high pressure and setting the timer to 20 minutes.
4. Use natural release method. Serve.

CHICKEN CHILI VERDE

This recipe needs 10 minutes to prepare, 30 minutes to cook, and it makes enough chili for 4-6 servings.

- Protein: 30.8g
- Net Carbs: 7.1g
- Fats: 32.5g
- Calories: 449

The macronutrient ratio of this meal is 6% carbs, 28% protein, and 66% fat.

INGREDIENTS

- Chicken Thighs and Drumsticks (3lbs bone-in, skin-on)
- Poblano Peppers (1lb seeds and stems remove, and chopped)
- Tomatillos (.75lb quartered)
- Ground Cumin (1 T)
- Jalapenos (2 with stems removed, chopped)
- Anaheim Peppers (2 with stems and seeds removed, chopped)
- Garlic (6 cloves, peeled)
- White Onion (1 C or 250mL, chopped)
- Fresh Cilantro (.5C or 125mL)
- Corn Tortillas
- Worcestershire Sauce (1 T)

INSTRUCTIONS

1. Set instant pot to sauté setting and combine chicken, peppers and spices in it. Heat until everything is gently sizzling. Seal the lid and then manually set it to high pressure before cooking your dish for 15 minutes.
2. Use the quick release method as per your manufacturer's instructions. Remove chicken and place in a separate bowl. Pour the remaining contents of your instant pot and all other ingredients you have left into a high-powered blender and blend everything until it comes together as a smooth, creamy gravy-style broth.
3. Remove bones from chicken, shred it, and then place it back in the sauce. Serve topped with fresh cilantro.

CHORIZO CHILI

This recipe needs 5 minutes to prepare, 20 minutes to cook, and it will prepare enough chili for 10 servings.

- Protein: 24g
- Net Carbs: 12g
- Fats: 22g
- Calories: 335

The macronutrient ratio for this recipe is 4% carbs, 48% protein, and 34% fat.

INGREDIENTS

- Bell Pepper (1 C or 250mL, chopped)
- Chorizo (2lbs)
- Onion (1 C or 250mL, chopped)
- Crushed Tomatoes (28oz can)
- Chilies (1.5 TSP, ground)
- Ground Cumin (1 TSP)
- Beef Broth (3 C or 750mL)
- Oil (1 T)
- Garlic Powder (1 TSP)
- Instant Coffee (.5 TSP)
- Cocoa Powder (.5 TSP)
- Black Soy Beans (15oz can, drained)

INSTRUCTIONS

1. Heat oil in instant pot over sauté setting. Brown chorizo sausage before adding onion and bell pepper. Cook until soft, then add spices to the instant pot. Allow it to continue cooking for a few extra moments until the spices are aromatic.
2. Once you can smell the spices, add the broth, tomatoes, instant coffee, cocoa and black beans.
3. Manually set your instant pot to the high pressure setting and allow your chili to cook for 10 minutes. When it is done, perform the quick release method recommended by manufacturer.
4. Serve.

SMOKY BACON CHILI

This recipe needs 15 minutes to prepare, 50 minutes to cook, and will prepare a total of 4 servings of chili.

- Protein: 28.2g
- Net Carbs: 10.9g
- Fats: 37.7g
- Calories: 515

The macronutrient ratio for this recipe is 9% carbs, 23% protein, and 68% fat.

INGREDIENTS

- Bacon (6 slices cut into 1-inch strips)
- Garlic (2 cloves, minced)
- Bell Pepper (2 C or 500mL, diced)
- Onion (1 C or 250mL, diced)
- Chili Powder (1 T)
- Ground Beef (1lb)
- Tomato Sauce (8oz can)
- Fire Roasted Tomatoes (14oz can)
- Garlic Powder (1 T)
- Cumin (2 TSP)
- Paprika (1 T)
- Cayenne Pepper (.5 TSP)

INSTRUCTIONS

1. Turn instant pot to sauté mode and sauté bacon until it becomes crispy. Leave fat in instant pot instead of using an alternative cooking oil for remaining part of cooking process.
2. In remaining bacon fat, cook onion, peppers and garlic. Sauté these ingredients until the onions become translucent.
3. Add remaining ingredients to the instant pot and mix thoroughly. Cook for an additional 5 minutes on the sauté setting before adding the bacon back to the pot.
4. Secure the lid on your instant pot and turn it to the Bean and Chili setting. If your instant pot does not have one, manually set it to medium pressure. Cook your chili for 30 minutes and then let your instant pot do a natural release on its own. When it's done, open the lid and mix your ingredients together well before serving.

TEXAS CHILI

This recipe needs 10 minutes to prepare, 15 minutes to cook, and it will prepare enough for 4 servings of chili.

- Protein: 30g
- Net Carbs: 12g
- Fats: 24g
- Calories: 395

The macronutrient ratio for this recipe is 4% carbs, 60% protein, and 37% fat.

INGREDIENTS

- Onion (1 C or 250mL)
- Ground Beef (1lb)
- Dried Oregano (1 TSP)
- Fire-Roasted Diced Tomatoes (8oz can)
- Oil (1 T)
- Ground Cumin (1 TSP)
- Garlic (1 T, minced)
- Chipotle Chilies in Adobo Sauce (1 T)
- Corn Tortillas (2)
- Water (.5 cup or 125mL)
- Mexican Red Chile Powder (1 T)
- Salt (2 TSP)

INSTRUCTIONS

1. Use sauté function on your instant pot to heat the oil and cook your onions and garlic. Cook until onions begin to soften before adding ground beef. Using a spoon, break up the ground beef and continue to cook it until it is browned.
2. In a blender, blend your tomatoes and corn tortillas until they are well combined.
3. In another bowl, combine your spices.
4. When beef is browned but not fully cooked, spice it with the spices in the recipe and allow it to cook for an additional minute, until the spices become fragrant. Add in the tomato blend. In the blender, add water and blend it to remove flavors from side of the blender. Then, pour the water mixture into the instant pot with the rest of your ingredients. Seal and manually set your instant pot to high pressure. Set the timer for 10 minutes and allow it to cook.
5. Allow your instant pot to naturally release before serving the chili.

TOMATILLO CHILI

This recipe needs 15 minutes to prepare, 35 minutes to cook, and it will prepare enough for 8 servings of chili.

- Protein: 20g
- Net Carbs: 6g
- Fats: 23g
- Calories: 325

The macronutrient ratio for this recipe is 2% carbs, 40% protein, and 35% fats.

INGREDIENTS

- Ground Pork (1lb)
- Ground Beef (1lb)
- Chili Powder (1 T)
- Tomato Paste (6oz can)
- Garlic Powder (1 T)
- Onion (.5 C or 125mL, chopped)
- Tomatillos (.5 C or 125mL, chopped)
- Jalapeno (1 T, chopped)
- Ground Cumin (1 T)

INSTRUCTIONS

1. Use the sauté function on your instant pot to brown your ground meats.
2. Once it's browned, add remaining ingredients to instant pot and stir thoroughly so everything is combined.
3. Secure the lid on your instant pot and manually set the instant pot to the high-pressure setting. Cook your chili for 35 minutes before allowing the pressure to naturally release.
4. When the release is done, serve your chili.

PART V

BEEF

Beef is a great meat that is filled with healthy nutrients such as iron. There are many great ways that you can cook beef to create flavorful meals that are a delight to eat. In this chapter we will explore the many different beef-based recipes you can make in your instant pot that are great for ketogenic dieters.

BEEF RIBS

This recipe needs 15 minutes to prepare, 35 minutes to cook, and it will prepare enough for 1 serving.

- Protein: 8.7g
- Net Carbs: 0g
- Fats: 0g
- Calories: 84

The macronutrient ratio for this recipe is 0% carbs, 100% protein, and 0% fats.

INGREDIENTS

- 3 cloves garlic
- 1 onion, quartered
- 1 tbsp olive oil
- 4 lbs/1800g beef short ribs

INSTRUCTIONS

1. Sprinkle ribs with salt.

2. Set to sauté. Add oil and allow to get warm. Brown ribs, after the oil, has heated.

3. Once ribs have been browned, place them in the cooker.

4. Add water, garlic, and onion.

5. Close and seal lid. Set on manual and cook for 35 minutes.

6. When finished, quick release the pressure.

7. Serve.

BALSAMIC BEEF ROAST

This recipe needs 15 minutes to prepare, 90 minutes to cook, and it will prepare enough for 1 serving

- Protein: 30g
- Net Carbs: 3g
- Fats: 28g
- Calories: 393

The macronutrient ratio for this recipe is 2% carbs, 67% protein, and 75% fats.

INGREDIENTS

- ¼ tsp xanthan gum
- ½ cup/113g chopped onion
- 2 cups/450g water
- ¼ cup/57g balsamic vinegar
- 1 tsp garlic powder
- 1 tsp black pepper
- 1 tbsp salt
- 3 lb/1370g boneless chuck roast

INSTRUCTIONS

1. Cut the roast in half. Season with garlic powder, pepper, and salt.

2. Set pressure cooker to sauté. Brown the roast on all sides.

3. Add ½ cup onion, 1 cup water, and ¼ cup balsamic vinegar to meat.

4. Cover and seal lid. Set on manual for 35 minutes.

5. When finished, release pressure naturally.

6. Open lid and remove meat. Shred with two forks and discard and fat.

7. Turn to sauté and bring liquid in bottom to a boil. Simmer ten minutes.

8. Whisk in xanthan gum. Add meat back in and gently stir.

9. Turn off heat and serve as you would like.

MOROCCAN BEEF

This recipe needs 15 minutes to prepare, 90 minutes to cook, and it will prepare enough for 1 serving

- Protein: 4g
- Net Carbs: 4g
- Fats: 20g
- Calories: 218

The macronutrient ratio for this recipe is 3% carbs, 8% protein, and 41% fats.

INGREDIENTS

- 1 tsp salt
- 4 tbsp garam masala
- 2 lbs/900g beef roast
- ½ cup/125ml sliced onion

INSTRUCTIONS

1. Slice onion into strips. Put in bottom of slow cooker.

2. Place the roast on top of onions. Add salt and spices.

3. Cover. Set on low and cook for eight hours.

4. Remove roast and shred with forks. Cook for another two hours to let the spices soak into the meat.

5. Serve with keto tortillas.

ASIAN POT ROAST

This recipe needs 5 minutes to prepare, 45 minutes to cook, and will make enough pot roast for 12 servings.

- Protein: 38g
- Net Carbs: 0g
- Fat: 9g
- Calories: 245

The macronutrient ratio for this recipe is 0% carbs, 63% protein, and 12% fat.

INGREDIENTS

- Boneless Chuck Roast (4-5lb size)
- Ginger (2 T, grated)
- Garlic (3 cloves, crushed)
- Orange Extract (1 TSP)
- Sugar-Free Fish Sauce (.25 C or 65mL)
- Granulated Sugar Substitute (such as Swerve) (3 T, divided)
- Water (.5 cup or 125mL)
- Red Wine Vinegar (1 TSP)
- Red Pepper Flakes (1 TSP, crushed)
- Orange Zest (1 T)

INSTRUCTIONS

1. Combine chuck roast, fish sauce, orange extract, garlic, 2 T of sweetener, ginger, water and red pepper flakes in your instant pot. Manually set it to high pressure for 35 minutes and allow to cook.
2. When done, use the quick pressure release method as outlined in your manufacturer's guide. Add remaining sweetener, orange zest, and red wine vinegar to the instant pot and stir.
3. Switch the instant pot to the sauté method and allow it to cook for an additional 5 minutes.
4. Serve.

BEEF STROGANOFF

This recipe needs 5 minutes to prepare, 30 minutes to cook, and it will prepare enough beef stroganoff for 4 servings.

- Protein: 33g
- Net Carbs: 9g
- Fats: 16g
- Calories: 321

The macronutrient ratio for this recipe is 3% carbs, 66% protein, and 25% fat.

INGREDIENTS

- Onions (.5 C or 125mL, diced)
- Garlic (1 T)
- Beef Stew Meat (1lb)
- Oil (1 T)
- Water (.75 C or 190mL)
- Mushrooms (1.5 C or 375mL, chopped)
- Worcestershire Sauce (1 T)
- Sour Cream (.33 C or 85mL)
- Corn Starch (.25 TSP)

INSTRUCTIONS

1. Begin by turning instant pot to sauté setting and melting oil. Sauté your garlic and onions until they are translucent.
2. Except for corn starch and sour cream, pour all remaining ingredients into your instant pot. Manually set instant pot to high pressure and cook for 20 minutes. Use the natural release method on your instant pot.
3. When the release is done, open the lid and stir in remaining ingredients. Turn the instant pot to sauté mode and continue stirring until everything is mixed and creamy.
4. Serve over cauliflower rice.

CORNED BEEF AND CABBAGE

This recipe needs 15 minutes to prepare, 1 hour 15 minutes to cook, and it will prepare enough corned beef and cabbage to serve 12.

- Protein: 23.7g
- Net Carbs: 8.1g
- Fats: 22.8g
- Calories: 334

The macronutrient ratio for this recipe is 3% carbs, 47% protein and 35% fat.

INGREDIENTS

- Corned Beef Brisket (4-5lb)
- Black Peppercorns (2 TSP)
- Dried Mustard (2 TSP)
- Cabbage (8 C or 2,000mL)
- Water (6 C or 1,500mL)
- Garlic (4 cloves)
- Onion (1 C or 250mL, sliced)
- Celery Stalks (1 C or 250mL, chopped)
- Carrots (1 C or 250mL, cubed)

INSTRUCTIONS

1. Place corned beef and water in the instant pot. Turn the instant pot to "Meat/Stew" setting, or manually set it to high pressure. Allow it to cook for 60 minutes.
2. Allow instant pot to naturally release before removing the lid, removing the brisket, and adding the vegetables. Keep the brisket warm while you cook the vegetables for 15 minutes on the "Soup" setting for your instant pot. When it's done, perform a quick release method as per your manufacturer's instructions.
3. Add beef back into the pot and choose warm setting to ensure all ingredients are at the same temperature before serving.

NO NOODLE LASAGNA

This recipe needs 10 minutes to prepare, 25 minutes to cook, and will make enough lasagna for 8 servings.

- Protein: 36g
- Net Carbs: 7.9g
- Fats: 3.2g
- Calories: 339

The macronutrient ratio for this recipe is 3% carbs, 72% protein, and 5% fat.

INGREDIENTS

- Garlic (2 cloves, minced)
- Onion (.5 C or 125mL, sliced)
- Ground Beef (1lb)
- Parmesan Cheese (.5 C or 125mL)
- Ricotta Cheese (1.5 C or 375mL)
- Marinara Sauce (25oz jar)
- Mozzarella (8oz, sliced)
- Egg (1 large)

INSTRUCTIONS

1. Begin by browning the beef and garlic in your instant pot using the sauté mode.
2. In the meantime, combine parmesan, egg, and cheese in a bowl until thoroughly blended.
3. Blend marinara sauce with browned beef, and then remove half of it. Spread a generous layer of about half of the mozzarella, then top that with the ricotta cheese mixture. Add back the remaining marinara meat sauce, then top again with mozzarella and then ricotta cheese. Finally, if there is any remaining, top it with the rest of your mozzarella slices.
4. To avoid condensation drips, put a layer of tinfoil over the lasagna before manually setting it to high pressure and cooking it for 8-10 minutes. This will help ensure that the cheese crisps. If you do not mind a runnier cheese, do not worry about this part.
5. Use quick release method, sprinkle additional dusting of parmesan cheese over the lasagna and let sit for about 10 minutes before serving.

PART VI
PORK

Pork is another staple meat when it comes to the ketogenic diet. Just as with beef, there are many great meals you can make that feature pork as the main dish. In this chapter you will explore a variety of pork-based meals that can be quickly created right in your instant pot.

FRITTATA

This recipe needs 10 minutes to prepare, 180 minutes to cook, and will make enough lasagna for 1 serving.

- Protein: 20g
- Net Carbs: 3g
- Fats: 16g
- Calories: 238

The macronutrient ratio for this recipe is 7% carbs, 8% protein, and 85% fat.

INGREDIENTS

- 1 1/3 cup/303g cooked breakfast sausage
- ¾ cup/171g frozen spinach, thawed, drained
- 1 tsp salt
- 1 ½ cup/340g bell pepper, diced
- ½ tsp pepper
- ¼ cup/57g diced red onion
- 8 eggs

INSTRUCTIONS

1. Combine sausage, pepper, salt, eggs, red onion, bell pepper, and spinach.

2. Pour into a greased pressure cooker.

3. Set on slow cook and cook on low for three hours until set.

4. Serve and enjoy!

KALUA PORK

This recipe needs 10 minutes to prepare, 120 minutes to cook, and will make enough lasagna for 1 serving.

- Protein: 36g
- Net Carbs: 0g
- Fats: 30g
- Calories: 415

The macronutrient ratio for this recipe is 0% carbs, 39% protein, and 61% fat.

INGREDIENTS

- 2 tsp salt
- 4 lb/1800g pork butt
- 1 tbsp liquid smoke
- 1 tbsp olive oil
- ½ cup/112g water

INSTRUCTIONS

1. Cut pork butt in half. Set to sauté.

2. Add oil and heat. When heated, brown the pork on all sides.

3. Turn off the pot. Add liquid smoke and water.

4. Place meat into the cooker. Sprinkle with salt.

5. Close and seal lid. Set on high and cook for 90 minutes.

6. When finished, release pressure naturally. Open lid.

7. Remove meat and shred. Discard any fat. Pour juices from pot over meat to keep moist.

8. Serve over riced cauliflower.

9. Enjoy!

RIBS

This recipe needs 5 minutes to prepare, 40 minutes to cook, and it will prepare enough ribs to serve 6.

- Protein: 38.9g
- Net Carbs: 3g
- Fats: 46.5g
- Calories: 586

The macronutrient ratio for this recipe is 2% carbs, 27% protein, and 72% fats.

INGREDIENTS

- Pork Ribs (5 lbs, cut into sections to fit in instant pot)
- Onion Powder (1 TSP)
- Erythritol (3 T, divided)
- Black Pepper (.5 TSP)
- Ground Coriander (.5 TSP)
- Garlic Powder (1 TSP + 1 T)
- Allspice (.5 TSP + .5 T)
- Red Wine Vinegar (2 T)
- Liquid Smoke (.25 TSP)
- Paprika (1 TSP)
- Water (.5 C or 125mL)
- Onion Powder (.5 TSP)
- Salt (1.5 T)

INSTRUCTIONS

1. Begin by seasoning your ribs with salt, 1 T erythritol, pepper, onion powder, paprika, .5 TSP allspice, coriander, 1 TSP garlic powder. Rub the spices in so they stick all over the ribs. Place all pieces into your instant pot.
2. Mix remaining ingredients in a bowl until well combined, then pour over your ribs as a sauce.
3. Manually set instant pot to the high pressure setting and allow your ribs to cook for 35 minutes, then use quick release method to release pressure and steam.
4. Serve & enjoy!

PORK ROAST

This recipe needs 5 minutes to prepare, 60 minutes to cook, and will prepare enough pork roast to serve 6.

- Protein: 39.5g
- Net Carbs: 0.7g
- Fats: 30.9g
- Calories: 451

The macronutrient ratio for this recipe is 1% carb, 36% protein, and 63% fat.

INGREDIENTS

- Pork Roast (2-3lb)
- Cauliflower (4 C or 1000mL, chopped)
- Onion (1 C or 250mL, chopped)
- Salt (1 TSP)
- Garlic (4 Cloves)
- Black Pepper (.5 TSP)
- Celery (1 C or 250mL, chopped)
- Coconut Oil (2 T)
- Portabella Mushrooms (1 C or 250mL, sliced)
- Water (2 C or 500mL)

INSTRUCTIONS

1. Place garlic, cauliflower, celery, onion and water into instant pot. Give it a stir before putting the roast in and sprinkling pepper and salt over top. Manually set your instant pot to the high pressure setting, and turn the timer to let your pot roast cook for 60 minutes.
2. When done, use the quick release method to eliminate pressure from your instant pot. Remove pork roast and, if desired, transfer into a preheated 400-degree oven for the remaining of the cooking process to create a crispier texture.
3. Meanwhile, all remaining contents from your instant pot should be placed into a high-powered blender to be blended until they form a smooth gravy-like puree.
4. Turn the pressure cooker to sauté function and melt your coconut oil. Sauté your mushrooms until they are soft. Pour vegetable broth over the mushrooms and continue cooking until the mixture thickens.
5. Serve pork with mushroom gravy on top.

PULLED PORK

This recipe needs 10 minutes to prepare, 1 hour 30 minutes to cook, and it will prepare enough pulled pork to serve 10.

- Protein: 35g
- Net Carbs: 3.8g
- Fats: 36.6g
- Calories: 497

The macronutrient ratio for this recipe is 3% carbs, 29% protein, and 68% fat.

INGREDIENTS

- Pork Butt (3-4lb)
- Beef Broth (1.5 C or 375mL)
- Olive Oil (.25 C or 75mL)
- Garlic (1 T, chopped)
- Ginger (2 TSP, grated)
- Spice Mix (2 T, any desired spices)

INSTRUCTIONS

1. Rub spices into pork butt generously so that it is well coated. Place in Ziploc bag and allow to marinate for a few hours, or preferably overnight.
2. Remove pork butt from Ziploc bag and placed in an instant pot that has been preheated to the sauté function with melted oil. Sear every side of the pork butt. Give it approximately 3 minutes uninterrupted per side to ensure it is properly seared as this will contribute to the flavor of the dish.
3. Add broth and bring to a gentle boil. Meanwhile, use a hard spatula to scrape up brown bits from the instant pot to mix into the broth. Again, this contributes to the flavor.
4. Manually set the instant pot to a high pressure setting and allow your pork to cook for 95 minutes. When the timer goes off, allow your instant pot to naturally release pressure until it is completely depressurized before removing the lid. Move the pork to a bowl and cover with foil. Rest it until the meat cools down to a manageable temperature and then shred it. Ensure it rests before cutting into it to avoid losing the flavor.
5. Serve.

BBQ RIBS

This recipe needs 10 minutes to prepare, 1 hour 360 minutes to cook, and it will prepare enough to serve 1.

- Protein: 35g
- Net Carbs: 3.8g
- Fats: 36.6g
- Calories: 497

The macronutrient ratio for this recipe is 3% carbs, 29% protein, and 68% fat.

INGREDIENTS

- 1 tsp salt
- 3 lbs/1.4kg spare ribs
- 1 cup keto friendly barbecue sauce

INSTRUCTIONS

1. Salt ribs and put in the slow cooker.

2. Add ½ cup barbecue sauce.

3. Cover. Set on low and cook for six hours.

4. Remove ribs and allow to cool. This step can be done the day before if you would like.

5. To finish ribs, add more barbecue sauce to ribs and place under broiler about 7 minutes per side. This will give the ribs a crispy exterior.

TANDOORI PORK RIBS

This recipe needs 10 minutes to prepare, 1 hour 30 minutes to cook, and it will prepare enough to serve 1.

- Protein: 25g
- Net Carbs: 2g
- Fats: 4g
- Calories: 160

The macronutrient ratio for this recipe is 2% carbs, 8% protein, and 85% fat.

INGREDIENTS

- ½ cup/112g favorite barbecue sauce
- 2 lbs/900g baby back ribs
- 1 ½ tsp salt
- 2 bay leaves
- 3 cups/700ml water
- 1-inch ginger, chopped
- 4 tbsp Tandoori Spice
- 5 cloves garlic

INSTRUCTIONS

1. Cut the ribs to fit into the pressure cooker.

2. Place them in the cooker as flat as possible. It is fine to stack them.

3. Add two tablespoons spice, salt, garlic, ginger, and bay leaves.

4. Add water to cover meat.

5. Close and seal lid. Set on high and cook for 22 minutes.

6. When finished, naturally release pressure.

7. Carefully remove ribs and place on cutting board.

8. Cool with foil and set for five minutes.

9. Pat dry and cover with barbecue sauce and more Tandoori spice.

10. Grill or broil for five minutes each side.

11. Serve.

PART VII
LAMB

Lamb is a flavorful, nutritious and hearty meat that can be used in many different ways. In this chapter you will learn about some incredible recipes that you can design in your instant pot that feature lamb as the main ingredient.

INDIAN KHEEMA

This recipe needs 5 minutes to prepare, 15 minutes to cook, and it will prepare enough Indian Kheema for 4 servings.

- Protein: 15.6g
- Net Carbs: 7.8g
- Fats: 40.4g
- Calories: 334

The macronutrient ratio for this recipe is 7% carbs, 14% protein and 80% fat.

INGREDIENTS

- Onion (1 C or 250mL, chopped)
- Ginger (1 T, grated)
- Cinnamon (3-4 sticks)
- Cardamom (4 pods)
- Cayenne Pepper (.5 TSP)
- Garam Masala (1 TSP)
- Ground Beef (1lb)
- Garlic (1 T, minced)
- Salt (1 TSP)
- Turmeric (.5 TSP)
- Cumin (.5 TSP)
- Ground Coriander (.5 TSP)
- Water (.25C or 75mL)
- Cooking Oil (1 T)

INSTRUCTIONS

1. Set instant pot to sauté function and warm oil. Add cinnamon and cardamom and let sizzle until fragrant. Add ginger, garlic and onion and cook until the spices become fragrant and the onions are soft.
2. Next, place your ground beef in the instant pot and begin to brown it as you break it up. Before it completely browns, add remaining spices and water.
3. Manually set your instant pot to the high pressure setting and allow for the contents to cook for 5 minutes. Allow your instant pot to perform a natural release of pressure before removing the lid to serve your Indian Kheema.

Lamb Shanks

This recipe needs 10 minutes to prepare, 1 hour and 30 minutes to cook, and will prepare enough lamb shanks for 4 servings.

- Protein: 37g
- Net Carbs: 8.8g
- Fats: 64.2g
- Calories: 791

The macronutrient ratio for this recipe is 5% carbs, 19% protein, and 76% fat.

INGREDIENTS

- Oil (1 T)
- Lamb (4 Shanks)
- Garlic (4 cloves, minced)
- Salt (2.5 TSP, divided)
- Tomato Paste (1 T)
- Onion (1 C or 250mL, minced)
- Herbes de Provence (1 TSP)
- Chicken Stock (1 C or 250mL)
- Red Wine (.5 C or 125mL)
- Diced Tomatoes (15oz can, reserve juices)

INSTRUCTIONS

1. Using the 2 TSP of salt, season lamb shanks and then place them in your instant pot that has already been heated to sauté function with vegetable oil. Sear each side of the lamb shanks, giving them about 2-3 minutes per side to get a nice brown color. Work in batches of 2 to avoid overloading the instant pot.
2. Add garlic, Herbes de Provence, tomato paste and onion to the instant pot and sprinkle with remaining salt. Sauté ingredients for five minutes before adding remaining ingredients. Scrape brown bits off of the bottom and stir in before sealing the lid.
3. Manually set your instant pot to the high pressure setting and allow your lamb shanks to cook for 40 minutes. You will want to use the quick release method when the timer is done. Use it as outlined by your manufacturer before removing the lid and serving your lamb shanks.

RICH LAMB

This recipe needs 10 minutes to prepare, 3 hours to cook, and will prepare enough for 6-8 servings.

- Protein: 35.9g
- Net Carbs: 1.1g
- Fats: 47.5g
- Calories: 583

The macronutrient ratio for this recipe is 1% carbs, 25% protein and 75% fats.

INGREDIENTS

- Tallow (.5 C or 125mL)
- Onion (1 C or 250mL)
- Celery (1 C or 250mL)
- Rosemary (.25 C or 75mL)
- Red Wine Vinegar (.5 C or 125mL)
- Salt (1 TSP)
- Beef Stock (4 C or 1000mL)
- Lamb Shoulder (4lb, bone-in)
- Pepper (1 TSP)
- Tomato Puree (1 C or 250mL)
- Mushrooms (.5 C or 125mL)

INSTRUCTIONS

1. Begin by heating instant pot to sauté setting. Add rosemary, tallow, onion, celery and garlic and cook for 5 minutes.
2. Add red wine vinegar, salt, tomato puree and pepper. Cook for an additional 5 minutes. Add beef stock and give a good stir to mix ingredients well.
3. Add lamb shoulder to the pot. If necessary, add more beef stock or water to completely cover the lamb shoulder. Boil the stock before securing the lid on the pressure cooker. Manually set your instant pot to the highest heat and allow to cook until steam begins to release from the pot. Then, reduce it to low pressure and cook for 2 hours. When it's done, allow the instant pot to naturally release pressure.
4. Remove the lid, stir ingredients and place the instant pot back to sauté function. Allow for it to sauté until there is only ¼ of the total amount of liquid remaining.
5. Remove the lamb shoulder from the instant pot and cut into bite-sized pieces before returning them back to the sauce. Serve with your choice of keto-friendly toppings.

PART VIII
CHICKEN

Chicken is a versatile meat that is full of protein and other great nutrients. It can be used in an endless amount of ways to create various flavors, textures, and meals in general. In this chapter you are going to explore a variety of chicken-based meals that can be cooked in your instant pot in minimal timing.

JERK CHICKEN

This recipe needs 10 minutes to prepare, 360 minutes to cook, and will prepare enough for 1 serving.

- Protein: 26g
- Net Carbs: 0g
- Fats: 4g
- Calories: 150

The macronutrient ratio for this recipe is 0% carbs, 52% protein and 47% fats.

INGREDIENTS

- 1 tsp pepper
- 5 chicken breasts
- 2 tsp garlic powder
- 4 tsp salt
- 2 tsp white pepper
- 4 tsp paprika
- 2 tsp thyme
- 1 tsp cayenne pepper
- 2 tsp onion powder

INSTRUCTIONS

1. Mix all spices in a bowl.

2. Rub each breast with spices and put in pressure cooker.

3. Close and seal lid. Set on slow cook on low and cook for six hours.

4. Serve with favorite side.

CHICKEN MASALA

This recipe needs 20 minutes to prepare, 20 minutes to cook, and it will prepare enough chicken marsala for 4 servings.

- Protein: 32g
- Net Carbs: 19g
- Fats: 27g
- Calories: 460

The macronutrient ratio for this recipe is 6% carbs, 23% protein, and 41% fats.

INGREDIENTS

- Chicken Breasts (1lb, boneless & skinless)
- Plain Greek Yogurt (1 C or 250mL)
- Lemon Juice (1 T)
- Ground Ginger (.25 TSP)
- Ground Pepper (1 TSP)
- Garam Masala (1 T + 4 TSP, divided)
- Garlic (5 cloves, minced)
- Tomato Sauce (15oz can)
- Paprika (.5 TSP)
- Salt (.5 TSP)
- Turmeric (.5 TSP)
- Cayenne (.25 TSP)
- Heavy Cream (1 C or 250mL)

INSTRUCTIONS

1. Cut your chicken into 1-inch cubes. Place them in a bag and marinate using yogurt, 1 T garam masala, black pepper, ginger, and lemon juice. Sit for at least 1 hour, but preferably overnight.

2. When you are done marinating the chicken. Heat the instant pot to sauté function and cook the chicken until all sides are cooked. Add all remaining ingredients into the instant pot, except for the heavy cream. Manually set your instant pot to the high pressure setting and adjust the time to cook your chicken masala for 10 minutes. You will want to perform a quick release as described by your manufacturer's guidelines.

3. Return the instant pot to sauté mode and choose the low heat option to avoid curdling the cream. When it has become warm, add the heavy cream to your chicken masala and stir frequently until the entire sauce becomes creamy in texture. Continue simmering for a few minutes until the sauce thickens and reaches a saucy consistency.

4. Serve over cauliflower rice.

GARLIC BUTTER CHICKEN

This recipe needs 5 minutes to prepare, 40 minutes to cook, and will prepare enough garlic butter chicken for 4 servings.

- Protein: 47g
- Net Carbs: 3g
- Fats: 21g
- Calories: 404

The macronutrient ratio for this recipe is 2% carbs, 27% protein, 38% fats.

INGREDIENTS

- Ghee (.25 C or 75mL)
- Garlic (10 Cloves, minced)
- Salt (1 TSP)
- Chicken (4 breasts, chopped)

INSTRUCTIONS

1. Layer all your ingredients into the instant pot, starting with chicken. Manually set the instant pot to the high pressure setting and turn the timer to cook your garlic butter chicken for 35 minutes. When it is done, execute the quick release method outlined in your owner's manual.
2. Shred chicken breast
3. Serve and enjoy!

ROTISSERIE CHICKEN

This recipe needs 5 minutes to prepare, 40 minutes to cook, and it will prepare enough rotisserie chicken for 4-6 servings.

- Protein: 23.7g
- Net Carbs: 4.4g
- Fats: 60.7g
- Calories: 669

The macronutrient ratio for this recipe is 3% carbs, 15% protein, and 83% fats.

INGREDIENTS

- Chicken (1 whole)
- Salt (1.5 TSP)
- Pepper (.5 TSP)
- Oil (2 T)
- Paprika (1 TSP)
- Onion (1 C or 250mL, sliced)
- Chicken Stock (1 C or 250mL)
- Garlic Powder (1 TSP)
- Lemon (1 half)

INSTRUCTIONS

1. Stuff the whole chicken with sliced onion and half of a lemon. Combine spices in a bowl and blend with oil so that they are easy to rub all over your chicken. Make sure you massage it in.

2. Preheat instant pot to sauté function before placing chicken in, breast-side facing down. Cook for approximately 5 minutes before flipping the chicken over and cooking the other side for an additional 2 minutes.

3. Add chicken stock to the instant pot and lock the lid. Manually set your instant pot to the high pressure setting and cook your chicken for 25 minutes.

4. Execute a natural release to carefully remove the lid and taking your chicken out of the instant pot. Let it rest for 5-10 minutes before cutting to prevent the flavor from being lost in the juices. When it is done sitting, cut it up and serve it with the remaining broth juices spooned over the serving.

PART IX
SEAFOOD

Seafood has many properties that other meats don't carry. For example, high traces of omega fatty acids. It is a great meat for those on the ketogenic diet to help keep you nourished and healthy. In this chapter we are going to explore instant pot recipes that feature seafood in them.

CREAMY SHRIMP & BACON

This recipe takes 5 minutes to prepare, 15 minutes to cook, and will make enough creamy shrimp and bacon to serve 4 portions.

- Protein: 17g
- Net Carbs: 3.5g
- Fat: 29g
- Calories: 340

The macronutrient ratio of this recipe is 4% carbs, 12% protein, 41% fat.

INGREDIENTS

- Bacon (4 slices)
- Salmon (4oz, smoked)
- Mushrooms (1 C or 250mL, sliced)
- Coconut Cream (.5 C or 75mL)
- Shrimp (4oz, shelled)

INSTRUCTIONS

1. Begin by slicing the bacon into 1-inch strips. Then, set your instant pot to the sauté function and cook them until there is no pinkness left but they are not starting to crisp.
2. Add the mushrooms and cook for an additional few moments, until mushrooms soften.
3. Add smoked salmon and cook again for an additional 3 minutes before adding the shrimp. Cook until the shrimp is done. When it is, you can add any desired salt and pepper and pour in your coconut cream. Cook for one more minute, or until the sauce thickens.
4. Serve.

SHRIMP WITH COCONUT MILK

This recipe needs 10 minutes to prepare, 10 minutes to cook, and it will prepare enough for 4 servings.

- Protein: 16g
- Net Carbs: 4g
- Fat: 12g
- Calories: 192

The macronutrient ratio for this recipe is 1% carbs, 32% protein, and 18% fats.

INGREDIENTS

- Garlic (1 T, minced)
- Shrimp (1 pound, shelled)
- Garam Masala (1 TSP)
- Salt (1 TSP)
- Ginger (1 T, minced)
- Unsweetened Coconut Milk (4oz or 125mL)
- Turmeric (.5 TSP)
- Cayenne Pepper (.5 TSP)

INSTRUCTIONS

1. Begin by mixing all the ingredients in your instant pot. Cover it with foil before closing the lid and sealing it.
2. Manually set your instant pot to the low pressure setting and turn the timer to cook your shrimp for 4 minutes. Execute a quick release on the lid once done, as described by your manufacturer's instruction manual. Stir ingredients and add more coconut milk if necessary.
3. Serve.

PART X
VEGAN & VEGETARIAN

If you are not a meat eater, fear not! There are still many incredible dishes that you can make that both honor the ketogenic diet and can be easily created in your instant pot. The following dishes are a selection of some of the best vegetarian and vegan ketogenic recipes that you can create in minimal timing. Please note that each one will have its appropriate dietary label next to it, so you can quickly determine whether it is vegetarian or vegan.

HARD BOILED EGGS

This recipe needs 1 minute to prepare, 5 minutes to cook, and will prepare enough hard-boiled eggs for 16 servings.

- Protein: 6.3g
- Net Carbs: 0.36g
- Fat: 4.8g
- Calories: 71.5

The macronutrient ratio of this recipe is 2% carbs, 36% protein and 62% fat.

INGREDIENTS

- Water (1 C or 250mL)
- Eggs (16 large)

INSTRUCTIONS

1. Fit your instant pot with the wire rack that came with it. Pour water into the bottom and then fit 16 raw eggs on the rack. If you cannot fit 16, fit as many as you can so they are tightly nestled in. You do not want them bouncing around.
2. Close your instant pot and manually set it to high pressure and cook the eggs for 5 minutes. Perform a quick release as per the instructions in your manufacturer's guide.
3. Fill a large bowl with cold water and place the cooked eggs into the water to rest for 5 minutes before peeling underwater.
4. Serve.

MASHED CAULIFLOWER

This recipe needs 1 minute to prepare, 5 minutes to cook, and will prepare enough mashed cauliflower for 4 servings.

- Protein: 10.7g
- Net Carbs: 7g
- Fats: 19.1g
- Calories: 251

The macronutrient ratio of this recipe is 11% carbs, 18% protein and 71% fat.

INGREDIENTS

- Cauliflower (1 large head, cut into chunks and core removed)
- Water (1 C or 250mL)
- Butter (1 T)
- Garlic Powder (.25 TSP)
- Chives (1 handful)

INSTRUCTIONS

1. Prepare your cauliflower to be cooked. Add the steamer basket to your instant pot, then fill it with water and cauliflower chunks. Close the lid and manually set your instant pot to the high pressure setting and set your timer to cook the cauliflower for 4 minutes.
2. Do a quick release as per your manual's guidelines immediately when the timer is done and carefully remove the cauliflower from the instant pot and transfer to a bowl.
3. In the bowl with the cauliflower, add butter and any desired seasonings. Mash or blend with an immersion blender until you reach your creamy smooth consistency.
4. Serve.

SPAGHETTI SQUASH IN GARLIC SAUCE

This recipe needs 5 minutes to prepare, 15 minutes to cook, and will prepare enough spaghetti squash for 4 servings.

- Protein: 1.5g
- Net Carbs: 13.8g
- Fat: 4g
- Calories: 88.6

The macronutrient ratio of this recipe is 13% carbs, 3% protein, and 11% fats.

INGREDIENTS

- Spaghetti Squash
- Water (1 C or 250mL)
- Garlic (4 cloves, minced)
- Salt (1 TSP)
- Olive Oil (2 T)
- Sage (.5 C or 125mL)
- Nutmeg (A dash)

INSTRUCTIONS

1. Prepare the spaghetti squash by halving it and removing the seeds. Fill the instant pot with water and place the spaghetti squash inside, skin down. If necessary, you can stack them on top of one another if both won't fit at once.
2. Seal the lid and manually set the instant pot to high pressure and cook for 3-4 minutes.
3. Stir together oil and spices. For best result, gently heat them in a pan on the stovetop while the spaghetti squash cooks as this will release the flavors of your spices.
4. Do a quick release on the instant pot according to your manufacturer's guide and then remove the spaghetti squash from the instant pot. Pour oil and spice mixture over the squash and mix well, pulling the squash off from the sides to create the spaghetti-like texture.
5. Serve.

PART XI
SAUCES

Just because you are eating the keto way doesn't mean you can't enjoy a selection of fine side dishes and sauces to compliment your meal and add to the variety on your plate! This chapter features a series of amazing side dishes and sauces you can make to increase the quality of your meal and add more flavor to your dish.

BLACK BEAN DIP

This recipe needs 15 minutes to prepare, 30 minutes to cook, and will prepare enough black bean dip for 24 servings.

- Protein: 8.3g
- Net Carbs: 2.5g
- Fat: 18.7g
- Calories: 201

The macronutrient ratio for this recipe is 5% carbs, 15% protein, and 80% fat.

INGREDIENTS

- Black Beads (1.5 C or 375mL, dried)
- Onion (1 C or 250mL, diced)
- Paprika (1 TSP)
- Garlic (4 cloves, minced)
- Jalapeno (.33 C or 90mL, diced)
- Sea Salt (.75 TSP)
- Crushed Tomatoes (15oz can)
- Vegetable Broth (1.75 C or 440mL)
- Cumin (2 TSP)
- Lime Juice (from 1 lime)
- Chili Powder (.5 TSP)
- Ground Coriander (.5 TSP)

INSTRUCTIONS

1. Thoroughly rinse your black beans before placing them in the instant pot. Add all remaining ingredients in and then blend thoroughly.
2. Manually set your instant pot to the high pressure setting and turn the timer to cook the bean dip for 30 minutes. Use the natural release method until the instant pot has released pressure over 10 minutes. When your instant pot has been releasing for 10 minutes, use the quick release method as outlined in your owner's manual.
3. Transfer contents into your blender and blend until creamy and smooth.
4. Serve.

SOUTHWESTERN SPICY SPINACH DIP

This recipe needs 5 minutes to prepare, 20 minutes to cook, and will make enough to serve 10 servings.

- Protein: 13.1g
- Net Carbs: 5.7g
- Fat: 22.3g
- Calories: 269

The macronutrient ratio for this recipe is 8% carbs, 19% protein, and 72% fats.

INGREDIENTS

- Spinach (1lb)
- Sour Cream (.25 C or 75mL)
- Half and Half (.25 C or 75mL)
- Tomatoes (3 medium, finely chopped)
- Garlic (5 cloves, minced)
- Ground Cumin (1 TSP)
- Cheddar Cheese (1 C or 250mL, grated)
- Mozzarella Cheese (1 C or 250mL, grated)
- Cream Cheese (4oz, cubed)
- Olive Oil (1 T)
- Onion Powder (1 TSP)
- Jalapenos (2, seeded and minced)
- Chili Powder (1 TSP)
- Hot Sauce (1 T)
- Black Olives (.5 C or 125mL)

INSTRUCTIONS

1. Begin by sautéing the spinach, garlic, and tomatoes in your instant pot. Cook until the spinach is cooked down and wilted. Turn off the instant pot.
2. Add all the dairy products, olives, jalapenos, hot sauce and spices into the instant pot and manually set it to high pressure and cook for 4 minutes. Perform a quick release of the pressure as outlined in your manufacturer's guide.
3. Season with salt and pepper if desired, then serve.

CHEESEBURGER DIP

This recipe needs 5 minutes to prepare, 20 minutes to cook, and will prepare enough cheeseburger dip for 10 servings.

- Protein: 8.3g
- Net Carbs: 2.5g
- Fats: 18.7g
- Calories: 201

The macronutrient ratio of this recipe is 5% carbs, 15% protein, and 80% fat.

INGREDIENTS

- Ground Beef (.5lb)
- Diced Tomatoes (10oz can)
- Cheddar Cheese (1 C or 250mL, grated)
- Cream Cheese (8oz, cubed)
- Water (4 T)
- Bacon (4-5 slices, cut into half-inch pieces)

INSTRUCTIONS

1. Sauté the bacon in your instant pot until it is cooked but not crispy. Place it on a paper-towel lined plate to rest for now.
2. Cook ground beef until it is completely browned, then add water, bacon and cream cheese into the pot. Do not stir the ingredients together, rather let them sit as-is.
3. Seal the lid and manually set the instant pot to high pressure to cook the dip for 4 minutes before performing a quick release as per your manufacturer's guidelines.
4. Add remaining cheeses and stir consistently until the cream cheese chunks have dissolved and the entire dip is creamy.
5. Serve.

PART XII
DESSERTS

Desserts can be tricky with the ketogenic diet, but there are still many great dishes you can end your meal with. In this chapter we are going to explore a selection of delicious desserts you can make in your instant pot. Note that these are ketogenic friendly, so you can comfortably make them without worrying that you are going to break your dietary requirements and exit the ketosis state.

ALMOND CARROT CAKE

This recipe needs 10 minutes to prepare, 50 minutes to cook, and will prepare enough almond carrot cake for 8 servings.

- Protein: 6g
- Net Carbs: 6g
- Fat: 25g
- Calories: 268

The macronutrient ratio for this recipe is 2% carbs, 12% protein, and 38% fats.

INGREDIENTS

- Almond Flour (1 C or 250mL)
- Swerve (.66 C or 170mL)
- Apple Pie Spice (1.5 TSP)
- Heavy Cream (.5 C or 125mL)
- Coconut oil (.25 C or 75mL)
- Eggs (3 large)
- Baking Powder (1 TSP)
- Walnuts (.5 C or 125mL, chopped)
- Carrots (1 C or 250mL, shredded)

INSTRUCTIONS

1. Grease a small cake pan. In a bowl, combine all ingredients until they are well-incorporated, but avoid over mixing. You want it to be light and fluffy. Pour in the greased pan and cover with foil.
2. Pour 2 cups of water into the inner liner of the instant pot and put a trivet in place. Fit the cake pan in your instant pot.
3. Cook on the CAKE setting for 40 minutes, then allow the instant pot to perform a natural release for 10 minutes before switching to the quick release method outlined by your manufacturer's guidelines.
4. Let it cool, then serve.

COCONUT ALMOND CAKE

This recipe needs 10 minutes to prepare, 40 minutes to cook, and it will prepare enough coconut almond cake for 8 servings.

- Protein: 5g
- Net Carbs: 5g
- Fats: 23g
- Calories: 236g

The macronutrient ratio for this recipe is 2% carbs, 10% protein, and 35% fats.

INGREDIENTS

- Almond Flour (1 C or 250mL)
- Swerve (.33 C or 85mL)
- Apple Pie Spice (1 TSP)
- Shredded Coconut (.5 C or 125mL, unsweetened)
- Baking Powder (1 TSP)
- Eggs (2 large)
- Heavy Cream (.5 C or 125mL)
- Butter (.25 C or 75mL)

INSTRUCTIONS

1. Begin by combining all the dry ingredients in one bowl. Combine the wet ingredients in a separate bowl. Pour the wet ingredients into the dry ingredients and combine well. The mixture should be light and fluffy, not dense.
2. Grease a small cake pan and pour the ingredients into it. Cover with a layer of foil.
3. Fill your instant pot liner with 2 cups of water and fit it with a trivet. Fit the cake pan inside of your instant pot and seal the lid.
4. Manually set the instant pot to high pressure and cook for 40 minutes. Allow the instant pot to perform a natural pressure release for 10 minutes before switching to the quick release method instructed by your manufacturer's guide. Open the lid.
5. Remove the cake from the instant pot and allow it to rest for 10-20 minutes before serving it with your choice of keto-friendly toppings.

DARK CHOCOLATE WALNUT CAKE

This recipe needs 10 minutes to prepare, 30 minutes to cook, and will prepare enough dark chocolate walnut cake to serve 6 portions.

- Protein: 8g
- Net Carbs: 7g
- Fats: 28g
- Calories: 301

The macronutrient ratio for this recipe is 2% carbs, 16% protein, and 43% fats.

INGREDIENTS

- Almond Flour (1 C or 250mL)
- Chopped Walnuts (.25 C or 75mL)
- Heavy Cream (.33 C or 90mL)
- Swerve (.66 C or 170mL)
- Baking Powder (1 TSP)
- Coconut Oil (.25 C or 75mL)
- Eggs (3 large)
- Unsweetened Cocoa Powder (.25 C or 75mL)

INSTRUCTIONS

1. Begin by mixing all dry ingredients in one bowl and all wet ingredients in another. Then, incorporate the wet ingredients into the dry ingredients and stir well so that the mixture is light and fluffy, not heavy and dense.
2. Grease a small cake pan and pour the cake mixture into the cake pan. Cover it with foil to avoid condensation falling on top of the cake and ruining it.
3. Pour 2 cups of water into the liner in your instant pot and fit it with a trivet. Then, fit the cake pan inside of the instant pot and manually set it to high pressure to cook for 20 minutes.
4. Allow the instant pot to naturally release for 10 minutes before using the quick release method outlined by your manufacturer's guide.
5. Allow cake to cool for 10-20 minutes before serving.

LEMON CHEESECAKE

This recipe needs 10 minutes to prepare, 40 minutes to cook, and will make enough lemon cheese cake for 6 servings.

- Protein: 5g
- Net Carbs: 2g
- Fat: 16g
- Calories: 181

The macronutrient ratio for this recipe is 1% carbs, 10% protein, and 25% fats.

INGREDIENTS

- Sweetener (.25 C or 75mL)
- Cream Cheese (8oz)
- Lemon Zest
- Ricotta Cheese (.33 C or 90mL)
- Lemon Extract (.5 TSP)
- Eggs (2 large)
- Sour Cream (2 T)

INSTRUCTIONS

1. Combine all ingredients except for sour cream and eggs in a bowl. Blend until it is completely smooth and free of clumps.
2. Add the eggs and blend until they are just incorporated. Do not overbeat or the cheesecake will not cook properly.
3. Pour the ingredients into a small greased cake pan and cover with foil to avoid the cheesecake being ruined by condensation.
4. Pour two cups of water into the inner liner of your instant pot and fit it with a trivet. Place the cake pan on the trivet. Manually set your instant pot to high pressure and cook for 30 minutes. Allow it to completely release the pressure naturally.
5. When it is done, remove the cheesecake from the instant pot and cover with sour cream while the cake is still warm, so it spreads on smoothly.
6. Put the cheesecake into the fridge and allow it to chill for 6-8 hours before serving.

THAI COCONUT CUSTARD

This recipe needs 5 minutes to prepare, 30 minutes to cook, and will prepare enough coconut custard for 4 servings.

- Protein: 6g
- Net Carbs: 6g
- Fat: 14g
- Calories: 174

The macronutrient ratio for this recipe is 2% carbs, 12% protein, and 22% fats.

INGREDIENTS

- Eggs (3 large)
- Unsweetened Coconut Milk (1 C or 250mL)
- Swerve (.33 C or 90mL)

INSTRUCTIONS

1. Begin by blending together all of the ingredients. Then, pour it into a heat-safe dish and cover the dish with foil.
2. In the inner liner of your instant pot, pour 2 cups of water. Fit it with a trivet, then place the heat-proof dish in the instant pot. Manually set it to high pressure and cook for 30 minutes. Allow the pressure to completely release naturally, do not use the quick release method. This is when the custard will set.
3. Remove the dish from the instant pot and allow it to come to room temperature before transferring it into the fridge. Allow it to cool completely until the custard is set.
4. Serve.

Made in the USA
Middletown, DE
14 December 2017